IT'S NEVER TOO LATE

Betty Scott

A Memoir

IT'S NEVER TOO LATE

Copyright ©2023 Betty Scott

ISBN: 979-8-9886760-1-0

All rights reserved. No part of this publication may be reproduced, distributed, or transmitted in any form or by any means, including photocopying, recording, or other electronic or mechanical methods, without the prior written permission of the publisher, except in the case of brief quotations embodied in critical reviews and certain other noncommercial uses permitted by copyright law. This also included conveying via email without permission in writing from the publisher.

Published by

Emerge Publishing Group LLC

Riviera Beach, Fl 33404

Printed in the United States

THANK YOU

To Sherry:

Thank you for being obedient from the time of your birth to now; your motherhood to the twins—Keith and Kai; your dedication to your career in nursing and working with me throughout the years; Continuing to be my daughter, girl-friend, DUE to my age— The support you give me. May God continue to bless you.

To Keith:

Thank you. Rather than pursuing a career in the medical field, you pursued your education as a business manager, and a radio personality. You are blessed with your speaking voice. Thanks for passing the state examination for Texas and Florida life agent. As a young child and now a grown man, a man of many principals, you respect the will of God as a man. As you mother, I can say THANK YOU SON. You have always had God's love for others. Thank you for your loyalty to your twin sister, Kai and your deep love for me. I deeply appreciate you.

To Kai:

As a young teenager, pursuing your goals, you worked at two large grocery stores. At the age of fifteen as a cashier, in West Palm Beach, Florida; one was Grand Union and the other Pantry Pride.

You received your Medical Assistant license from New England Tech and helped me in the medical field. You have had many accomplishments. I complement you for being my daughter and twin to Keith; for growing up with your brother, putting up with him when you were young with your first car. He rode all the gas out of the car then brought it back to you empty. When tires were needed, he bought cheap tires. You were loyal to your brother with much love. Now your loyalty is shown to me.

THANK YOU FOR YOUR ASSISTANCE WITH ME WHEN NEEDED. MAY GOD BLESS YOU.

To Trina:

God bless you Trina, for your loving dedication to your marriage, and your success to your organization with action sports recreation center. You have a great ability to work with young people, as well as your family. Your son is blessed to have a Mother that is a Mother to your needs. I also want to thank you for your deep seeded love and concern for your husband and how you two worked together. You both are blessed to have each other. MAY GOD BLESS YOU AND YOUR MARRIAGE.

To My Grandkids:

I thank all of you—grands and great grands— for being in my life. Each one of you has been inspirational and joyful to my life. I am not finished with my career until I see each one of you graduate and become a successful person. I am looking forward to Niyah's graduation in 2024. I am grateful for my precious one, Makaia, who comes at my beck and call at the age of 13; may God bless me to see her graduate in 2028. I am very grateful for her love, and devotion to me, her grandmother, Betty Scott. I offer many blessings to Chantel wherever she is. She graduated from Hampton University; she is a Docter of physical therapy, I shall never forget this blessed day on mother's day May 12, 2019. God blessed me to attend her graduation. My prayers are with all of my grandchildren.

TABLE OF CONTENTS

Chapter 1	Detroit was Hot	11
Chapter 2	Growing Up	13
Chapter 3	My Community	15
Chapter 4	No Comparison	17
Chapter 5	Brother Petty	19
Chapter 6	My Sister Bea	21
Chapter 7	My First Flight	23
Chapter 8	Undecided	25
Chapter 9	Guess What!	27
Chapter 10	Faith	29
Chapter 11	Chicago	31
Chapter 12	Marriage	33
Chapter 13	Newly Weds	35
Chapter 14	My First Born	37
Chapter 15	My Second Child	39
Chapter 16	10 Years Later	41
Chapter 17	The Biggest Surprise	43
Chapter 18	Awaiting	45
Chapter 19	The Arrival	47
Chapter 20	My Older Children	49

Chapter 21	Nursing Course	....	51
Chapter 22	Weekend Trip	....	53
Chapter 23	The Ram in the Bush	....	55
Chapter 24	No Return	....	57
Chapter 25	Rich and Famous	....	59
Chapter 26	Returning Home	....	61
Chapter 27	A Distraction	....	63
Chapter 28	Plans Made	....	65
Chapter 29	From Detroit to Florida	....	67
Chapter 30	307 Foresteria Drive	....	69
Chapter 31	Love One Another	....	71
Chapter 32	Tragedy	....	73
Chapter 33	From Nurses to Family	....	75
Chapter 34	Betty Jane Scott	....	77
	The Family Tree	....	78
	Ackacknowledgements	....	81
	The Scott Companies	....	83

CHAPTER ONE
DETROIT WAS HOT!

The city of Detroit, Michigan is the largest in the mid-western state of Michigan. It was settled in 1701 by rich colonists. There are many stories about Detroit, Michigan. One of my favorite Detroit stories in particular is about the great Henry Ford.

Henry Ford was the founder of Ford Motor Company, and chief developer of the assembly line technique of mass production.

Ford created the first automobile that middle-class Americans could afford. Henry Ford built his first Model T car in 1908. He became world famous after selling millions of cars. Later in the book you will find out about my father working for Ford Motor Company. Detroit is also known as Motor City Capital. Many talents were discovered there such as Aretha Franklin, Diana Ross, Smoky Robinson, Gladys Knight, and many more.

I can't forget Berry Gordy, producer of many talents. Berry was born November 28, 1928. He was born three years before me. He is now 94 and I turned 92 on October 8, 2023.

People are always asking me what my secret is to making it to my 90's. First, my faith in my Father, my love for others, my steadfast faith and always taking my toils and snares to God in prayer.

CHAPTER TWO
GROWING UP

I was born October 8, 1931 and grew up in a small village north of Detroit, Michigan. My mother delivered me at home, which was 372 La Belle Street; Highland Park, Michigan. This was many, many years ago. I grew up in Highland park. When I reached the age of five, I was enrolled in kindergarten. My education continued through high school.

I was introduced by Ma to the quality of life. I was taught the importance of respect. In those days I dressed like a teenager. I never knew of or owned a pair of blue jeans. It was dress or slacks with decent shoes supporting my arch. A purse was a must, with lace gloves when attending an event; a hat when going to church. This is the way it was.

In those days there were no shopping malls. My family had no car; they only had papa's truck. We had to travel by street cars catching the street car on Woodward Avenue. It would take us straight down Woodward Avenue to all the big stores. Also, there was the great FOX THEATER which opened in 1928 and closed in1980. Then there was the Paradise Theater which opened Christmas day, 1941.

Many of our great orchestra bands performed there until 1951. it was a lovely place to go to enjoy our great musicians. I was old enough to enjoy the bands of Duke Ellington, Count Basie, Ray Charles, Louis Armstrong and others.

DETROIT WAS HOT!

I graduated at the age of 17. This time I felt like I was a grown up so I got a job in downtown Detroit. During those days, this was the area where my mother had introduced me to our etiquette shopping at JL Hudson Department Store. I was intrigued with the well-dressed elevator operators with white gloves, black tailored dresses, and their hair neatly styled. When she took me shopping this was my favorite store.

When it was time to apply for a job, I applied at Kerns Department Store, Crowley's, Annis Furs, and many more stores. Annis Furs was my pick because it was part-time and seasonal. The job consisted of calling their customers to pick- up their furs to be placed in storage for the summer months and then delivered in the fall or winter. All merchandise was tagged and checked for cleaning or repairs. This was a very interesting job to me since I like to talk. I fit in well with this job.

My parents were disappointed that I didn't continue college. In my mind I knew this job was going to be a season for my future, and that is what I meant.

My parents were born in the south. Mother was from Cookeville, Tennessee and daddy was from Nashville, Tennessee. They were truly southerners. Somehow, they got together and dated, became serious and decided to move to Michigan.

I would love to know more about their courtship, but my mother was a very private person. She didn't talk about events concerning her life. That was just her personality.

I began thinking that was old fashioned; I would always be happy to discuss my beautiful life with my children.

CHAPTER THREE
MY COMMUNITY

In our community was all races: African American, Jews, Chinese, and Polish people.

As a child growing up, this part of my life I will never forget. As I write this book at the age of 92, let me stop and praise the Lord for my ability to be able to write my second book. The first book was published in 2012. The title of the first book is Can't Cut the Mustard.

The first book was a guide for loving God's people. Now I will continue writing this book.

In our neighborhood three houses down was a neighborhood grocery store owned by a Jewish couple, Mike and Tracy. They had hearts of gold. The store was very small, but they managed to find room for their stock including all kinds of assorted candy, squirrels for one penny, tootsie rolls for one penny, and Baby Ruth for a penny. A penny went a long way; so did a nickel and a dime.

My mother had credit with them, not a credit card; it was a little yellow book with data, and price of purchases. Her agreement was to pay once a month on the outstanding balance.

My parents didn't have to worry about food and household products. it was a blessing not having to rely on food stamps or apply for food stamps. In my day I think people received a book of stamps which were coupons. Today they have credit cards.

We lived in a neighborhood that was full of beautiful homes and manicured yards. It was a community where everyone knew every family. Many activities were performed at our churches as well as the YMCA. Children grew up with both parents. My mother was a housewife. Jesus was a big deal in our family and we were taught to pray at all times.

On Sundays we went to Sunday school, early church services and evening service. On Easter and Christmas we had a program where we had to recite a skit or poem. I was brought up in the church. Ma cooked every Saturday and Sunday. Sometimes she would invite our pastor and his wife for dinner.

As you can see there was no time in my life to be disobedient. It is hard for me to see and tolerate children today due to the lack of guidance they get from their home.

CHAPTER FOUR
NO COMPARISON

My father was one of many that worked on the assembly line for Ford Motor Company for many years. He also had a part time job. This part time job was in the evenings. He would come home get in his truck and go searching for junk. He searched for old furniture such as tables, chairs, cabinets and things that were usable or maybe needed little repair. Then he sold it to different individuals.

Daddy was all man, a man of integrity. He didn't want mother to work; he felt her place was to be home taking care of the family. This also gave her time to attend school meetings, church meetings, and prayer meetings. Mother also had her own daily routine. Her mornings were dedicated to reading one chapter in the Bible. Prayer was very important in our home, and it still is in my life. That is what the world needs— more prayer and faith in the world, and most of all love!

In the world that I lived in many years ago we had peace, love, and happiness. We could leave our doors open in the summer months when the weather was hot and sleep by the windows and doors.

There is no comparison to our life today. You dare not leave a door or window open. An alarm system is definitely needed today.

CHAPTER FIVE
BROTHER PETTY

My brother was older than I. We had very little in common. He and his friends would get together and play basketball, but very little football.

I was grateful to him for looking out for me. When his friends were around me, I was protected from them getting fresh with me. His name was John Petty and my name before marriage was Betty Jane Petty. I never got upset about it to this day. I thought it was very cute.

My brother took up a trade after high school. He went to barber school and became an outstanding barber.

There was a friend of the family that owned a barber shop in Highland Park, Michigan on the main street called La Belle. The corner of La Belle and Lincoln was where the young boys hung out just to talk, have fun looking at the girls, and talk trash. There was never any fighting.

A few steps away was the barber shop where my family got Petty a job. He had his own private barber chair and did very well cutting the hair of young boys and men. He had a humorous, loving, and honest personality. Petty had many friends as well as lots of girlfriends. He finally married and had his first child—a boy named Tyrone Petty. Then two more little Pettys came along—Terry and

Toya. I still remember playing with them. I was young and they stayed with Ma.

Ma played a big part in our lives. The only thing was Ma could keep secrets. Apparently, Petty had an affair with a young girl and she became pregnant and had a baby out of wedlock. The young girl confided in Ma. One day she visited Ma and brought a picture of the baby boy. Ma immediately hid the picture. She took it upstairs and hid it. I've never seen the picture to this day.

Later, I was told who the boy was. I am his aunt. I was told that Petty was a rolling stone. There is a lady living that is my niece. I talk to her occasionally. I was born at a time when it was disgraceful to have a baby out of wedlock.

I missed out of knowing many relatives in my family. God blessed Ma. She did the best she knew how.

CHAPTER SIX
MY SISTER BEA

My sister, Buenola, was a Petty until she married her first husband, Melvin Byous. Bea was a High school graduate. Her beauty and her interest was her hair and different hair styles. She enrolled in beauty school and cosmetology. She became a hair dresser.

Bea was a very glamours lady and very independent. She decided after graduation she would travel. Her first destination was Philadelphia, Pa. She made many friends in Philly. Next, she was off to New York where she met and cultivated friendships that lasted for many years.

My sister never forgot me. She always sent me letters, cards, gifts, and money. To me she was a great sister.

Bea never had children. She did very well in Philadelphia. She had her own Beauty Salon. She met many popular people that could benefit her with her business.

In the 1900s beauticians who worked on black folks hair, worked extremely hard due to our many types of textured hair— nappy, kinky, tightly curled, unstraightened hair.

To those that don't know about the straightening comb, the hair had to be separated into small parts of the hair. It was then combed and straightened with a hot comb. Many years of this pulling and use of your hands along with standing in one spot using your back with no support could cause one to seek early retirement. So this was Bea's case. She retired after many years of this hard work pressing and hot curling hair. She never had the opportunity to perm hair. Perms can be traced back to 1872. The perms we see today weren't invented until 1938; I was 7 years old. I didn't have pressed or permed hair until I became a teenager. Of course, people have a choice today between the curling irons and the perms. I'll take the perms any day for my hair .

The world has changed in many aspects. Thank God I am still alive and here to talk and write about the beautiful life that I am living. If you are unattractive and need or want hair of any color, money will buy your needs ; whether you want eye lashes of any length or fancy nails. So you see, beauty is in the making.

CHAPTER SEVEN
MY FIRST FLIGHT

My sister, Bea, returned back home to Highland Park. During the years Bea had moved to Philadelphia, my family had moved to 45 Kendall in Highland Park, Michigan. This house was much bigger than our last one. It had three bedrooms with an upper level. Although we moved, we were still in the same neighborhood

I still had my part time job downtown at Annis Furs. After the season of my job, my sister wanted me to go on a short trip with her to Cleveland, Ohio. She wanted me to meet this couple in Philadelphia. It appeared to me that Bea liked to show me off to her friends. it was odd because I often wonder about her always sending me gifts. I realized this was a sister with a kind heart, but what about Ma? She should receive some blessings sometimes from her.

I enjoyed my first flight to Cleveland, Ohio. Bea and her friends enjoyed taking me sightseeing. During that time I wasn't 21 yet so I was too young to go to the bar. My sister and her friends wanted to go have a drink in the bar before dinner so they took a chance and took me into the bar. Everything went well. They had alcohol drinks and they ordered me a Shirley Temple. What an exciting experience for me.

I started to become fearful of what Ma would say if she knew I was in a bar, but that's not all I saw. I also saw a young man behind the bar that was attracted to me. He appeared to be enjoying looking at me. He asked me what my name was, where was I from, and how long I would be staying in Cleveland. I replied and gave him the particulars. What a lovely trip. I was so ecstatic and happy and I was hoping I would hear from this tall handsome man one day.

CHAPTER EIGHT
UNDECIDED

After my trip with Bea, I decided I would take a course in nursing to become a certified nursing assistant and nurse. I decided to continue working at Annis Furs until I could enroll in a nursing program. I began realizing I had to have a degree in order to live a rich life, and to be independent enough to take care of myself.

My sister and brother have done very well with their trades, so I can't give up with my dreams and future. My future is more important to me than getting excited over the first man that looks good to me. Everything that glitters is not gold. I also knew Ma would be disappointed in me if I didn't further my education. I always wanted Ma to be proud of me. It was hard because she was from the old school—very strict, and old fashioned. Later in my life, I am grateful that she was strict because she made a respectful lady out of me.

CHAPTER 9

GUESS WHAT!

Guess what! When I came home from work, mother said "Betty, you had a call from some man from Cleveland. He asked to speak with you. I told him you were not at home and asked if he wanted to leave a message. So hear is your message."

"Oh! My God, he wants to visit me."

My mother's head dropped. "Where did you meet this man?"

"Ma, I met him in Cleveland, Ohio when Bea took me to visit her friends."

" Well, she didn't tell me."

"Ma, again I repeat, I am of age to date."

"Yes, but I just can't help it. I guess I am old fashioned."

" Yes, you are. Please trust me Ma, I would never hurt you, so just relax. You will met him. The man's name is ELLIOTT SCOTT."

He really worked fast calling me. I have to accept the call and visit. It was a beautiful week end. I was impressed with him. He was well dressed well-coordinated and looked good in his clothes. It appeared to me he could be a sweet loving person, but a little conceited because he was a fine honk of man.

He wined and dined me and we had so much fun together. The weekend flew by fast. He stated he had moved to Chicago and took a job in sales and he would like to give me a trip to visit him.

"Would you like to visit me and see Chicago?"

" Well, I will have to think about this beautiful offer. Please call me when you return home. We have so much to talk about."

"I will," he stated.

I never said to much about him after he left for Chicago to Ma or Bea.

I couldn't wait to talk to my girlfriend at work about my weekend with Elliott. When we got a chance to talk, my friend could hardly wait to hear about my week end with Elliott.

"Girl, he is fine, 6ft 3ounces, tall, light brown skin. His hair was a very good grade in other words, good hair."

"Betty, you hit the jack pot."

"All I can say is he is handsome and fine. He is working fast. He wants me to visit him"

"Where"?

" Girl, all I can say is don't move too fast."

CHAPTER TEN
FAITH

I began thinking and reliving the beautiful weekend that I had with Elliott. I was trying not to think negative about him. Why did I fall for a man that lives in another city? Oh well, I have to pray about this relationship. "

This is what Ma taught me. You have to always put GOD into your life and pray about all things that come into your life. Why? Because prayer changes things, that is if you have the faith. I have the faith so I will take him up on a trip to see him in Chicago. At this point, I had not heard from the nursing program so I will get ready to visit Elliott. When I return from my trip, I will pursue the requirements of nursing school. I also should find out more about Elliott's back ground. He did tell me he served in the army, active duty. He had a scar on the side of his lip. It wasn't that noticeable. His father and mother had died early. He had cousins and a host of friends in Akron, Ohio. It seemed to me he likes to travel. So, I will see the outcome. Falling in love is beautiful but can be HELL.

CHAPTER ELEVEN
CHICAGO

Elliott said he had already made arrangements for me to stay with his landlady's friend who lives around the corner. Her name is Priscilla Brown. His landlady's name is Joy Baker. It appeared to me that he was as excited as I was. The fact that he had made arrangements for me to be comfortable and safe, told me he was all man. We really have to get acquainted, that is, if possible. I would love to see as much as I can of Chicago.

Elliott didn't have a car so getting around was difficult. We used the L transportation, street car, public transportation. Remember, this was in the 1950's not 2023. I enjoyed the L ride. It took us down town to State street where many elegant stores were. Unfortunately, we didn't do any shopping but we did a little sight-seeing.

Elliott hailed a cab. This is how he was accustomed to getting around. In those days, I didn't drive and if I did, I wouldn't drive in Chicago. I got a chance to meet some of Elliott's friends. It was important for me to know the company he was keeping. He had a friend that was in the Army with him. They had remained friends. His name was Brown. He was a licensed Barber for years. The barber shop where he worked for years was on 63rd street on the south side of Chicago. I got to see this busy neighborhood with many businesses. We had lunch at one of the neighborhood restaurants on 63rd street. Mr. Brown appeared to be a lovely man and a good friend.

CHAPTER TWELVE
MY MARRIAGE

I found myself wanting to marry Elliott before he proposed. I felt he had good standards for a man, and he had fallen in love with me. Elliott made plans for me to ship my clothes and my personal things to Chicago. All plans were made and paid for by Elliot. We were married at the Justice of Peace in Chicago Illinois.

I was 21 years of age; Elliott was in his thirty's, ten years older than me. The age difference was something to think about. Well, it is too late to think about it. Oh well, we are in LOVE.

CHAPTER 13
NEWLY WEDS

The first year of our marriage was exciting. We lived with Mrs. Baker. She made us very comfortable until Elliott found us a two-bedroom apartment on the south side of Chicago on 83rd Street. Elliott had applied for a manager's job at MARY JANE SHOE STORE on 63rd street in Chicago, Illinois. He was blessed to get the job. He was one of the first Blacks to my knowledge to work for this company. Sixtty-third Street was all business. I began learning my way around, and I talked to Elliott about my getting a job. He stated, if that is what you want to do that is fine with me, but make sure it is a day time job.

Since I knew my way on the L transportation, I went to State Street downtown. While walking around I saw a Fur Store. Having worked at Annis Furs, I went into the fur store and applied for the same description of a job I had at Annis Furs and was hired the same day

I was happy to see how independent I was growing up to be in such a big city. I was blessed with a job the same day. Elliott appeared to be happy for me. We had very little social life since we both were working. We enjoyed our time together.

"How is your family?" asked Elliot. "I like talking to your sister."

"Why do you ask?"

"Because you never talk about them."

"Well, I love them but Ma didn't approve of me getting married. She wanted me to continue college. I disappointed her but maybe one day I will further my dream in nursing."

"Perhaps if you give her a call often and get to know her, you both will come around. Ma is set in her old fashion ways."

" Betty, we will visit them soon."

" I would love that. "

CHAPTER FOURTEEN
MY FIRST BORN

I have a surprise and what a Surprise!

"Elliott, I think I'm pregnant."

"You what? I've never been accused of fathering a child in my whole life."

"Well, I have an appointment with the gynecologist."

Elliott's statement didn't bother me. It wasn't nice but I expected it because it is what it is. It appears Elliott has a little selfish and jealous streak about me with people. I was a little disappointed about him not being excited like I was. The best thing for me to do was take it to the Lord and pray.

Elliott was not a man of God. He grew up with no father, a sick mother and no siblings. He showed signs of selfishness. This is what I saw with that statement. I noticed that he doesn't like me to converse to long with Mrs. Baker. Oh well, he is my husband.

After coming from the Docter, all I remember to this day was being pregnant with my first child, a boy weighing in at seven pounds, eleven ounces. He was very healthy. We named him after his father, Anthony Elliott Scott. We both were very happy and after a few months of him being born things changed.

We decided to pack up and move to Detroit where the family could enjoy our first child and we would be one happy family.

We stayed with Ma while I was away in Chicago. Ma had met her a man and he moved in. My sister moved downtown Detroit. I remember the street— Garfield and John R. During those days and years, downtown Detroit was a spot to party. My sister loved the elegant style. To be flattered was up her alley. As for Ma, if she was happy with her husband, I have to go along. Everyone needs somebody and my father was no longer living.

CHAPTER FIFTEEN
MY SECOND CHILD

We started all over again. We stayed with Ma until we found a house in the suburbs and we rented it. We were lucky. Elliott got a job at s Department store on Grand Blvd managing the shoe dept. I became a full-time housewife.

Tony was a hand full and soon would be a year old. By that time I was pregnant again. Elliott took the news with a happy attitude. He stated "I hope it's a girl so Tony and her can grow up together." "Well," I said, "We have to be grateful for what God gives us."

Thank God Elliott's concept has changed. March 25, 1956, I gave birth to a girl. She was eight pounds, four ounces, a big healthy baby girl. Compared to Tony, she was an easy baby to care for. I was able to keep her on schedule with her baths and meals. She was such a peaceful baby and to this day she is a joyful, peaceful, caring, and loving person.

As time went by, we entertained the children with games, pets, and visits to the park. Sunday school was always on a Sunday. Tony was a real lover of fish and turtles. We had a small aquarium for each one.

They were children who were very happy at home with different activities. Sherry loved to play house with her brother and sometimes they had different programs on our black and white television that they watched. Thank God in their days of growing up there were no cell phones. Remember, this was 1954 to 1956. And as I write this book, I am 92 years of age. I pat myself on the back to be able to remember the highlights of my life.

CHAPTER SIXTEEN
10 YEARS LATER

Years passed by. We enjoyed watching our children grow up without a thought about having more children.

Surprise! Surprise! I was pregnant again. It had to be nine or ten years after our first children were born.

The Doctor confirmed my pregnancy. I waited a few months into my pregnancy to tell my family. This time Elliott stated " Well damn. What is going on?"

I said, " A BABY."

"Elliott said "I can't believe it; this is crazy."

"Baby, do you think I'm happy with nine months of being fat and uncomfortable?"

The only thing that made me feel better was that the children were happy. As for Elliott he will get over it; after all he is the father.

This pregnancy was very different and difficult in my fifth and sixth month. I had such a weakness with doing my house duties. I waited for my check up with my Docter. The doctor said, "Betty, you are fine, but I will have you take an x-ray. We will call you to give you a report."

Each day I was no better. The children felt so sorry for me. It was so cute. They began learning how to clean, and wash. We didn't have a microwave so I didn't encourage them to cook. They enjoyed learning how to clean and do household duties.

They asked, "Mom, are you happy to have us help with the house?"

"Yes."

I was so uncomfortable. "I have an appointment with the gynecologist tomorrow."

"Good, we hope all goes well with our brother or sister."

CHAPTER SEVENTEEN
THE BIGGEST SURPRISE

It was the biggest surprise. I arrived by bus to the Doctor's office. I was sitting in the lounge waiting to be called. The Doctor walked out said, "Come with me. There is a reason why you feel so weak. Sit down. You have two babies in that stomach."

"What? Two babies?"

"Yes," said the Doctor.

"I can't believe it."

"One baby is very high. The other one is right under. Your stomach is very full. The babies look good. So take it easy. Eat small portions. Take your vitamins. Rest when you feel weak or tired."

"Thank you, doctor. I am speechless." I walked out of his office in a daze.

"Lord, what will I do?" The Lord didn't answer. I had to get myself together and catch the bus home.

Sitting on the bus, in my mind I was trying to get my mind together to tell Elliott and the children the news. I think I will stop at my neighbor's house and tell them the great news. Perhaps their response will help me tell Elliott and the children.

When I told the neighbors they said, "Are you kidding?"

"No, I am not. I just left the Doctor's office. The x-ray showed I am having twins."

"Oh wow, how wonderful, two babies. Go girl! You are something else."

"Yes, I am. After ten years the children will be excited. I don't know how Elliott will take it. I will let you know how he takes it. He is not a candidate for more children. See you later. Thank you for being happy for me."

"Hi honey, how was your day?"

"Fine."

"How did it go at the doctors today?"

"You better sit down," I answered.

"Betty, what is going on?"

"Well, we are having twins."

"Did you say twins?"

"Yes twins, as I said two babies is twins. Thank God, no more than two."

Elliot asked, "Where are we going to put all these babies?"

"Don't be silly," I told him.

"They will be in bassinets until they get of size then we have to get beds. In this case, let's take one day at a time; they haven't arrived yet."

"Ok, mommy dearest," he said.

CHAPTER EIGHTEEN
AWAITING

While waiting for the big surprise, nothing much has changed. My period of weakness continued as well as a fullness in my upper stomach. I was almost bedridden at that time. I told myself there was no reason to complain; it will be over soon.

This had to be a gift from God and it was a big one. The children helped me pack my little suitcase. They were so happy.

"I want a sister," said Sherry.

"I want a brother," said Tony.

"What do you want mother?"

"I just want them to be healthy, I'm sure." I felt like a trunk. Elliot had no comments about baby names or anything. He just wanted to get the show on the road.

That night my water broke. "OH HELL, LETS GO BEFORE YOU HAVE THOSE BABIES," said Elliot.

"Elliott, give me a minute. I have to put my toothbrush, comb, and brush in my bag."

Elliot yelled, "BETTY, LETS GO BEFORE YOU HAVE THOSE BABIES HERE!"

CHAPTER NINETEEN
THE ARRIVAL

We arrived at the hospital very late at night. My doctor was called. In those days delivery was performed in the operating room. Today you have a private room. The nurse was prepping me. When my doctor arrived the show was on.

Baby number one, a boy came right away. Baby number two was a girl. She wasn't ready yet; it took 30 minutes for her to come out. She was breeched, meaning her position was wrong. Her head was up instead of down. In those 30 minutes, she moved around and the Docters were able to assist in her delivery.

I was so glad that during those 30 minutes I was sedated. Waiting that long there was no telling what would have happened to me, but overall I had great Docters. No wonder I was so uncomfortable. Baby number one was five pounds. Her brother was taking up all the space in my stomach.

That was a big experience. I tip my hat to any mother who has to experience giving birth to two or more babies.

Elliott and the children and myself had names for both babies before they were born. All we had to do is confirm their gender. The girl, Kai Buenola Scott; the boy, Keith Earl Scott.

We were disappointed that Kai had to stay in the hospital longer due to her not inhaling that much oxygen. In a way this was good;

it gave us a little more time to get everything organized with the baby supplies. We had to purchase cases of diapers. Everything had to be in large quantities. We were lucky my family gave me a baby shower before the birth of the babies. I remember one gift, the sterilizer that disinfected the bottles; it ran 24 hours a day .

Diapers were washed daily. No pampers. It was fun and the family enjoyed the twins different personalities growning up.

CHAPTER 20
MY OLDER CHILDREN

After a week we brought Kai Home. Not only did the older kids stay busy assisting with the care of their sister and brother, they had discussed their names for the twins.

SHERRY said " I will take the boy and his play name will be DIPPEST.

Tony said "Well, I will take the girl and her play name will be Janie.

I said, "You both have it all figured out. Remember, they are not dolls; they are infants, real people. Be careful with them. I will show you how to care for them."

Elliott was very quiet throughout all the planning, enjoying a glass of scotch and soda. I guess he needed something for his nerves.

Sherry and Tony were 10 years older than the twins. Growing up they were very private children who played with each other.

There was a concern about Tony. He was very smart but he would stay away. I could hear him talking to his turtles. He trained two to have a race. I never knew you could train turtles. Well, I guess I found out you could train turtles. This didn't mean he had a problem; he was just a very private person. They both enjoyed being home trying to get back to the twins to meet their needs. I never asked them to do anything for the twins. They were always on time even with the poop! I am very happy that my older children have compassion and love for one another to this day. Sherry and Tony were excellent baby sitters as well as very meticulous with our home. They became the best cleaning people you could ever have.

CHAPTER TWENTY-ONE
NURSING COURSE

Since the babies were doing so well and almost six months old, I felt I could go out for a few hours. This was the time for me to look into a course in nursing. In the years of the fifty's it was called Nurses Aid. Later, it developed into a course that qualified one to be a Certified Nursing Assistant. My first goal was to get certified.

First, I had to talk to my husband, second my built in baby sitters. The family agreed for me to further my education. Tony and Sherry were very interested in the course. They would ask questions along with tutoring me. I was very happy when I received my certification. Time was going by fast. The twins were growing up.

We had to think about a larger home. Blessed by the best—God. We were able to purchase a three- bedroom home in the City on the end of Linwood and Puritan. I still remember the address, 16176 Linwood and Grove There is a school at the corner where Keith and Kai went to elementary school.

Our neighbor was a teacher at an elementary school downtown. She had grandchildren that were enrolled at her school. We became very supportive of each other. She suggested that Keith and Kai enroll at her school.

I talked it over with the family. Their daddy agreed since there are more opportunities at her school.

"Yes," I stated. "Keith is interested in football and they have a program for sports."

"Good."

We settled that. After the change of school they received so much knowledge, traveling back and forth to school. To this day the twins are 57 years of age. Big Ma, my neighbor, left a prayer with them:

I AM HAPPY, I AM HEALTHY, I AM SUCCESSFUL. TODAY IS THE GREATEST DAY OF MY LIFE,

AND TOMORROW WILL BE EVEN BETTER.

This prayer is often prayed by Keith and Kai.

CHAPTER TWENTY-TWO
WEEKEND TRIP

I had met a very nice lady at school. We talked about going for our LPN license. We started the course and we studied and did our home work together at my home. Things was going well. I was surprised when Elliott said he wanted to visit his home in Akron, Ohio for the weekend.

"Yes, that would be nice. When will you return?"

"Perhaps Sunday night or Monday."

"Good. Me and the children will spend the weekend going to church and dinner."

To this day, I don't understand why he didn't return. He could have had an accident, or he could have died, or something could have happened to him. I thought he was happy!

When he finally called, he was in Chicago. I couldn't listen to his story or his lies. My focus was on how I would make it. Elliott had done such a beautiful job supporting us with all our needs. He was short on his fatherly duties with the boys, such as activities with the boys, such as sports, fishing, and homework. He was not good at explaining life to our children or having a relationship with them. In other words, he didn't know how to express his love to them.

He didn't know Jesus. There was jealousy within our marriage. I suspected it in our early marriage. Perhaps I should have discussed the problem with him instead of putting it under the table. Who knows the minds of others. It was very difficult for me. I had to remember GOD always has a ram in the brush.

CHAPTER TWENTY-THREE
THE RAM IN THE BUSH

I had to be strong. There was no time to be sad. I had to talk to the older children. "Your father is not in Akron; he is in Chicago. I hate to say he told a lie."

"Why would he tell a lie?"

"Your guess is as good as mine. All I know is the show must go on."

"We will help you mother."

"Thank you, children."

Perhaps this is why I had these beautiful children with so much love and hearts of gold.

"We will make it with the help of our Lord and Savior. Let us pray!"

I put all my faith in one person and that is not man, but GOD. I believe in what I said. Faith is what I have.

I will never forget our yellow telephone on the wall. It rang that same evening. "This is Mrs. Scott. Who's calling?"

"I have a Patient in my Convalescent Home that is looking for a private duty certified nurse for five days on the day shift. Would you be interested?" OH, my God. I answered, "Yes."

She gave me the address and appointment was made. Everything went well. It was my friend that recommended me for the job. I started on a Monday. That gave me one weeks salary.

I found time on my lunch hour to call about my bills—the Detroit Edison Light Company, Gas company, Michigan Bell, my mortgage company. I found each one due. How devastating. This man must have gone crazy and left me for no reason. I could never trust him in our life again.

This is when I went to work with the support of Sherry and Anthony better known as Tony. I worked day and night. I would go home and check on my children, taking food and orders on a notepad—do's and don'ts that reflected on the job and their duties.

The children carried out all their duties. I had to adjust without Elliott. I never felt sorry for him due to him lying to me and if he could do it one time, he will do it again or break my heart as well as the children's heart.

The twins had to be between 11 and 12 years old. Sherry and Tony were older. I had the opportunity to get Sherry into the nursing field by her taking a course in assisted nursing at a convalescent home. I was blessed to take a case in a private home in Detroit in the summer, and winter in Florida. This meant I had to leave the convalescent home. I had to do what was best for me along with the pay that was excellent.

In taking the job, I was asked to get a relief so this gave me an opportunity to train Sherry. This is when we started to work together. Sherry was 17 years old. Everything worked out with the twins because they were reliable. Throughout all my toils and snares God has been with me.

CHAPTER TWENTY-FOUR
NO RETURN

Elliot soon returned back to Detroit. What do men do after they have left you? They beg you to take them back. Well, HELL NO! just that fast I applied for my divorce.

Elliot couldn't believe it. Instead he believed I had another man. He's the one who had another woman in Chicago. After he dined with her and gave her everything and God knows what else, she was done with him. He should feel like an asshole. We had been married 18 years and he lost his cool. All I can say is he was a fool and you never know what is in the minds of a person. After Elliot got the message, he went home to Akron, Ohio. We really didn't communicate anymore and I didn't have time to make him pay child support. Why? Because while I was at the child support office listening to other mothers cursing about their husbands not paying child support for their child, I could work and stay ahead instead of begging and not getting a dime. No child support or food stamps for me. I am doing just fine, or shall I say faith is my blessing and I turned 92 on October 8th, 2023. I never heard of someone dying from work.

CHAPTER TWENTY-FIVE
RICH AND FAMOUS

It was in the summer when I started this case with a wealthy couple. They had a cook, maid, a chauffeur and now a nurse for her husband 24 hours a day 7 days a week. I worked the day shift. Sherry worked the night shift. I had to brief Sherry about the day as well as the night shift.

"Sherry, when you come on duty read your notes first."

"Yes, I will Mother."

"Betty, do you think you could go to Florida with us and stay until I get a nurse in Florida?

Without a doubt or question I answered "yes."

"This will be in October depending on the weather. If it gets cold here, we will go earlier" stated Mrs. Goldberg.

October came. The preparation began. It was very interesting getting ready for Florida. Mrs. Goldberg ordered three large cartons for clothes. The car was packed with things that were needed in Florida. The chauffer left before us. The maid and cook cleaned the apartment after we left as well as checked on the apartment until we returned.

The three of us traveled first class. I was wearing a black dress and black swede boots, never thinking about black appears hot. I was really hot. Never again will I wear a wool dress and swede boots.

When we got off the plane the heat hit me. I thought I would burn up. The chauffer greeted us. Driving from the airport, Mrs. Goldberg briefed me on all the sights, going across the first bridge.

The beautiful Palm Trees, were in bloom when we arrived to their Florida apartment. What a beautiful apartment! Looking out the sliding patio door, there were beautiful sculptures and flowers. I made myself comfortable and got out the hot clothes I had on. I made my patient comfortable.

Mrs. Goldberg asked the chauffer to take me on Country Road to show me the main highlights and the great Publix stores. She also talked about the baked goods, and the produce. She loved the whole store.

In the late 1900's, the store was small. After some years it became larger. Then there was Green's Drug Store with a fountain that served breakfast and lunch. I heard many movie stars met there to have breakfast together, and talk trash.

The drug store was owned by two brothers and had been there many years. Medications and other supplies were ordered from this drug store. Across the street is a big catholic church where the Kennedys attended church. The post office was also in the area. So far, I was good. I could walk from their apartment and shop.

CHAPTER TWENTY-SIX
RETURNING HOME

We were very busy unpacking. Mrs. Goldberg said she had to hire a cook and a nurse.

"Betty, I want you to evaluate the people and I will do the rest."

"Thank you. I will."

Everything worked out while I was leaving the Goldbergs in the hands of their Florida staff. I said to Mr. Goldberg, "I enjoyed my trip; it was like a vacation."

"Betty, how much do you owe me?"

We laughed. He had got to know me so he was joking with me.

"Mr. Goldberg, I will see you in Detroit."

My flight was safe and the children were glad to see me. The children briefed me on all the news. We always enjoyed our home and work together.

"Would y'all like to move to Florida?"

"Moving to Florida is what brought this on." stated Anthony.

The twins asked, "What will we do with our belongings?"

"Children think about it. Because I have made up my mind. It is a great opportunity for us, no cold weather plus a better opportunity for the twins to complete school plus Detroit is starting to get rough.

So when winter comes, I will go with them and work with them until they return back to Detroit. This will give me the opportunity to get us a house or apartment. I realized we would have to get new furniture because our furniture is too heavy to be brought to Florida. I planned to have a yard sale and sell most of our belongings.

"Children, don't worry. I have it all planned. Sherry, if you and Tony wish to stay in Detroit you can."

"Oh no. We will go with you," stated Sherry."

"Ok, so I will rent or sell our home."

The twins were around 13 or 14 years old. They were old enough to make their own decisions.

CHAPTER TWENTY-SEVEN

A DISTRACTION

Oh! MY God.

"Ma, what is it?"

"I just received a call. Your father is in the hospital in intensive care. Oh my! What shall I do?"

There was an undesirable feeling running though my body. Keith wanted to go see about his father. So I made arrangements for Keith and I to fly to Akron. I had never been to Akron. It was awkward for us so we went directly to the hospital. All information was given to me. We went into his room. Keith called out to him, " DAD."

He opened his eyes. "I told those people not to call my family."

I said to myself, he still has that arrogant way on his death bed. I felt sorry for Keith. After all, that was his father. I could see that time was of the essence. I did manage to get his home address and key to his apartment. We went to his apartment. We met his neighbor; she was very nice and helpful. I decided that Sherry and Tony should see their father, so I made arrangements. Kai was in college so she didn't go.

I spent all my savings. I felt it was the thing to do for our children. The last visit I made arrangements with a funeral home for cremation, sending ashes home for a memorial service. It was sad that Elliott had a beautiful life with us. It was senseless to think looking for love in the wrong place when love waited for him at home. He also denied his health with Diabetes. He was dying with many other complications. He had no life insurance. He had put God on the back burner of the stove. I pray that this is a lesson for his children.

It was a successful memorial service with the family showing love.

CHAPTER TWENTY-EIGHT
PLANS MADE!

Now that we have weathered the storm, we can start working on preparation for moving to Florida. I feel it in my gut; this beautiful move to Florida is going to be a success in our life.

We began preparation for our yard sale. Plans were made on a Saturday before I started working for the Goldbergs when they returned from Florida. This gave me time to get organized with the sale and renting the house out, and to find a dependable person to drive my car and bring the children to Florida. My plan was to tell the Goldbergs I was moving to Florida when they come home. Some of the members of my family made nasty remarks about the move.

One of my nosy neighbors took it upon herself to come to the house and asked me, "Are you crazy, moving to Florida? The Goldbergs would fire you." I said to her, "We will be just fine." She appeared to be very disgusted with me. I wanted to say something very nasty to her, but I didn't. She's just an old hag.

I hold all faith, not in man or woman, but in our Father, who art in heaven

CHAPTER TWENTY-NINE
FROM DETROIT TO FLORIDA

On the return from Florida I was glad to start my work with the Goldbergs. After they returned, I told them they wouldn't have to worry about traveling again due to me moving to Florida with my family.

"I have a reliable person driving my car and bringing my children."

Mrs. Goldberg stated, "That is wonderful. We will help you as much as possible."

"First when we return to Florida, I will rent a house or an apartment, and after renting it the children will come."

Everything went from Detroit to Florida. I found a beautiful house. The twins were also enrolled in a new school. Tony was working in a convalescent home. Sherry was working with me. Everyone was comfortable and happy.

Tony came up with a plan. He wanted to start a cleaning service, cleaning private homes, and also employing people to help. He also dreamed of a foundation to help feed and clothe the poor. The cleaning service was a great success.

During his business with Scott's Cleaning Service, he employed many young people and taught them how to clean. He had approximately 200 customers. His business lasted for many years until employees started stealing sodas and watches, and dresses. This is when people and personality started to change.

Tony became disgusted and started to become close to God. Somedays, he would lock himself in his room, reading the Bible. He started to lean on the Lord. This is when God started to come into his life.

He was affiliated with our Bishop and his minister friend. His friend was responsible for leading him to became ordained. He was baptized in January 2005 and licensed as a minister of the gospel of Jesus Christ. His trial sermon was delivered in August 2005, in Fort Lauderdale.

His ministerial goals were to reach the unsaved by deeds and example; to feed the hungry, and clothe the naked. He was a minister of the sick. He provided shelter to help the homeless and help someone to be able to help themselves. God delivered him from alcohol and drug addictions. God blessed him with spiritual gifts, intercessory prayer warrior and prophesy. He was a self-made man and was happy to have a relationship with God, the father and the Son. He found a father in God.

CHAPTER THIRTY
MY FAMILY SECRET

My sister and I were driving around looking for property in Riviera, Beach Florida because we thought property was cheaper than Lake Park Florida. The Spirit came over me and commanded me to go to Lake Park. There you will find a house for sale for Home Away from Home.

My granddaughter went to school at Lake Park Elementary in our neighborhood. I picked her up at the corner of 3rd Street and Foresteria Drive. There was a large sign HOUSE FOR SALE 307 Foresteria Dr. What a coincidence. I immeadialy turned the corner to Foresteria Drive which is the street where we live. We got out the car and peeked in the window. i could see it was just what I was looking for. This was in 2001. I called the realtor and she came right out. Right then we negotiated all papers. It wasn't long after that. In 2001 HOME AWAY FROM HOME was mine. I had to go through many inspections and a class every year. I received my license from Tallahassee. Again my family supported me.

Growing up, I always had a question in my mind. The concern, the giving, the complete love that my sister gave me was different than a sister. My sister's friends and relatives would make statements like "the older you get the more you look like your mother."

My mother, Yes. As I grew older and started putting things into perspective, I thought about how my sister could talk about her cousins to Ma. When I asked Ma anything about them, and asked if I could visit them. Ma would flat out and say "NO."

"They are not your cousins," stated Ma in a harsh voice.

I talked to my children "Could it be true that my sister is my mother?"

"Yes, mother. She had you very young. Look at your birth certificate. You were born at home ninety-one years ago in Detroit, Michigan, a suburb 372 La Belle Highland Park, Michigan."

It was an old birth certificate. In those days no telling what and how things were done. It was a disgrace to have a child in your early teens. Ma had to be embarrassed and kept it a secret. Only Bea's friends and cousins knew that she was pregnant and kept it a secret. If you continue lying about anything you start to believe the lie statements about BETTY JANE. I was told by Ma that they were no relation to me, so I guess they believed the lie. The good part about the lie is no matter who birthed me and where ever and whoever has never had any effect on me. I am still living a full life of joy, happiness, taking care of my sister or mother or whoever she is to me.

Due to Bea's age and condition she was Diagnosed with Alzheimer's. She was in our life and I had to take care of her. She had no children, so she said. Bea was blessed to have a home provided by me with love and dignity. August 12, 2003 at the age of 86 Bea departed from HOME AWAY FROM HOME. She was my sister or my mother.

During the time she was transitioning, my cousins and her closet friends kept calling me. "Did she tell you?

"Not yet." No, She died and to this day the question remains unanswered.

I did my part with all my heart and love.

CHAPTER THIRTY-ONE
LOVE ONE ANOTHER

Moving On In Life

Changes were made at Home Away From Home. I kept my certified nurse to run my business. She was very dependable and she did a wonderful job with my sister. I had decided to take a private case. This was supposed to be a short case and it lasted eleven years, taking care of a woman and her brother. Sherry worked with me throughout this case.

This case was a great experience to me. It was my first education. I learned how race can affect a person covered up by a person that has been raised with prejudices that continues being two-faced with their old antique ways. They cannot accept the fact that there is no difference in your skin and your race. White is white, black is black.

Black does not rub off on you. It is your heart, a clean heart that turns your attitude to have a loving heart, to accept any person or persons regardless of their color.

We were finally accepted after many changes; love stepped in. To this day I often think about the person whom I grew to love. Her presence is still with me. She encouraged me to write my first book CAN'T CUT THE MUSTARD. I never thought or imagined I could write a book. This is my second book: IT'S NEVER TO LATE!

The brother finally excepted CHRIST though the right way—accepting black people. This is deep when the brother asked God to forgive him from all of his sins. GOD TOOK HIM IN HIS SLEEP. May he rest in peace.

His sister continues to accept the fact of losing her brother. Sherry and I continue to give her love and she appeared happy. She also had a loving family. My friend lived on to be in her 90's.

CHAPTER THIRTY-TWO
TRAGEDY

I decided to semi retire and enjoy life in my little house that GOD gave me. My children stayed in the big house. Tony had his little house in the rear of a big house in Riviera Beach, Florida.

We have always had a great loving and giving family and throughout our life we worked together. As we grew older our love increased for one another. Tony was the oldest. He had many dreams and goals. His last dream was to preach the gospel and he dd that. He detoured many young people from drugs. It was his desire to have a foundation to feed the hungry, clothe the naked, and house the homeless. Some of his dreams went with him November 3rd. 2011. We celebrated his birthday with him that evening having dinner together, at the Cheese Cake Factory in City Place in West Palm Beach, Florida. I dropped him off at home around eleven P. M. never thinking this was my last time being with my loving son!

Around 5 P. M. there was a loud knock at my door. I was alone!

"Who is it?"

"The police! The police."

"You have the wrong address and person."

Then the police flashed Tony's picture on the window. That was my son. I opened the door.

"Sit down," the officer said. "Your son is dead."

"OH! MY! GOD. I left him early at home. What Happened?"

"A fire broke out in the kitchen and it expanded fast. Your son was taking his bird out to the yard along with his Bibles and many other personal things. 911 was called. He died on the way to the hospital. He inhaled too much smoke."

From that moment I cannot write or express what my feelings were. MY SON WAS DEAD! HE WAS GONE!

I found comfort in prayer and my faith. That's what got me though this tragedy. Tony was a believer and often talked about his FATHER IN HEAVEN. I am sure he went to heaven to be with his HOLY FATHER.

The viewing of my son was the answer to my grief and prayer. He looked like an Angel—peaceful. His hair was like silk, his skin like a baby. He was reincarnated. I walked away rejoicing. I know my son is in heaven so I live happy, not sad about the accident and his death.

My son left here knowing God the Father and the Son.

His words remain in my heart. "Mom. You've been my strength, the rock on which I stand. I've gained so much wisdom guided by your gentle hand. The kindness you have shown in every word and deed has been a blessing in my life in so many times of need."

CHAPTER THIRTY-THREE
FROM NURSES TO FAMILY

Sherry and I continue working together with the same patient. We had developed a close relationship with the family. Holidays were spent with the entire family which was our family. Sherry and I enjoyed making lovely holiday dinners for the entire family. We became more than nurses and to this day we remain the best of friends.

This is when Sherry became interested in baking Cakes with caramel icing. The Caramel icing was very difficult to make, but good. It is hard to get it to thicken, but she has the patience to make it. Then there is the pound cake that melts in your mouth. The pound cake is now her best seller. Baking cakes is Kai's hobby along with nursing.

CHAPTER THIRTY-FOUR
BETTY JANE SCOTT

I am having a blessed life, and I am fortunate to be so healthy and peaceful. My mind is still sharp and I have an excellent memory. I continue to stay active. it has been a pleasure writing my second book "It's Never Too Late."

It has given me a sense of joy along with entertainment and reminiscing over my life and getting the answers about my life. Life is real. I have accepted the good and the bad because life is what you make it to be. This is a book of wisdom. Always set a goal for yourself— the good and the bad. I stay busy reading, writing, craft work, making jewelry, cooking, cleaning, and a little driving to the grocery store, drug store, cleaners, and the bank. I enjoy church on Sunday. I also enjoy a once-a-year trip to visit my daughter-in-law and son in Texas.

As you read "It's Never Too Late" remember it's about prayer, wisdom, and faith. Be careful what you speak out your mouth. I speak to my brain about what I want to do " Betty get out of that chair and get busy." if I have a hard time getting up, I say "one, two, three" and keep on pushing. I am also blessed to have made it to my 92nd birthday October 8, 2023.

I have truly enjoyed my career and I miss my career but I realize I still have my career to complete. Remember, it's never too late. May God bless you.

The Family Tree

CHILDREN

Anthony Elliot Scott

Sherry Anita Scott

Keith Earl Scott

Kai Buenola Scott

GRANDKIDS

Anthony's kids

Anthony Scott II

Danielle Scott

Chantal Scott

Keith's kids

Austin Scott

Jordan Scott

Taylor Scott

Kristen Elise Scott

Kai's kids

Ellen Jane Hall

Ericka Janae Hall

Kaila Marshelle Hall

Makaia Denise Williams

Great Grandkids

Isabella Scott

Eniyah Hall

Johnathan Elliott Smith

Maurion Lymon

Anthony Hall

Jakai Johnson

K'iore Monae Johnson

ACKNOWLEDGEMENTS

A Beautiful Flower
By
Betty Scott

Thinking of a beautiful flower!

I want the flower to grow,

and be a healthy flower;

Knowing without food and water,

It will not be healthy and it will die.

*****

I thank my Father, Son, and the Holy Ghost for

caring, sharing, and loving me throughout my journey.

For many, many years, I give thanks to my first child

Anthony Elliot Scott born November 3, 1954. Thank God, he was born to be a husband, father, and son, with an unusual love for me. Before Anthony died, he left me with words of love: "Mother your heart is filled with love, for everyone you know, you ask so little for yourself it is time for your goodness to be proclaimed for all the world to see and hear. There is no mother more loved than you, my mother dear"- Anthony Scott

Now your loyalty is shown to me . Thank you for your assistance to me when needed. MAY GOD BLESS YOU.

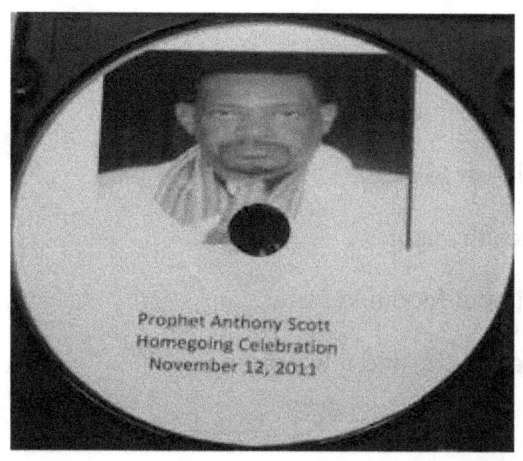

THE SCOTT COMPANIES

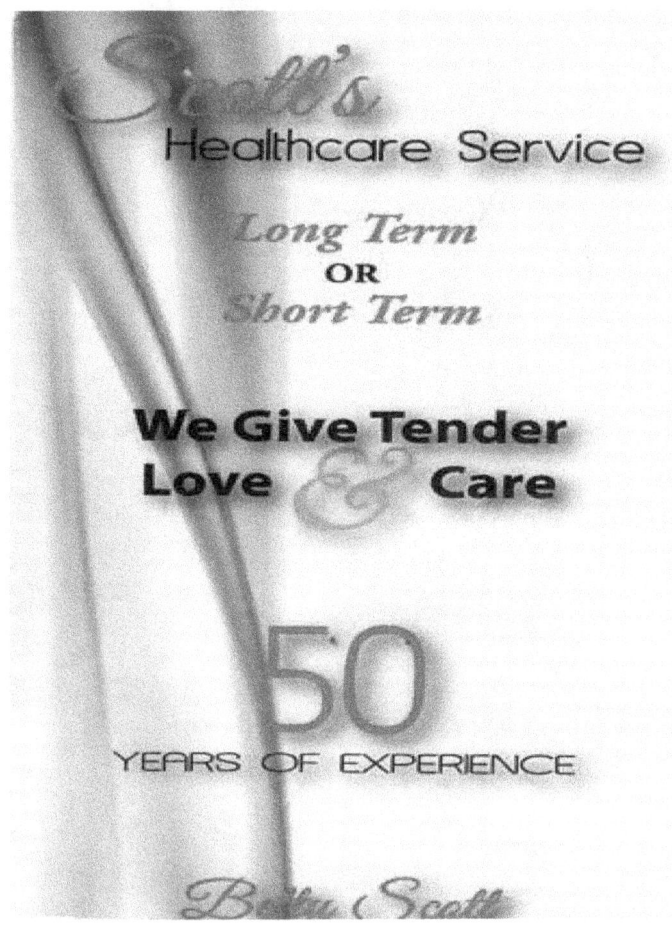

SCOTT'S CLEANING SERVICE

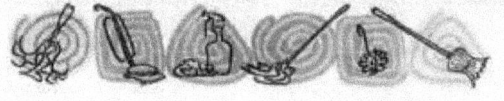

"For Service that's a must, and Service you can trust, Don't delay, call Scott's today"!

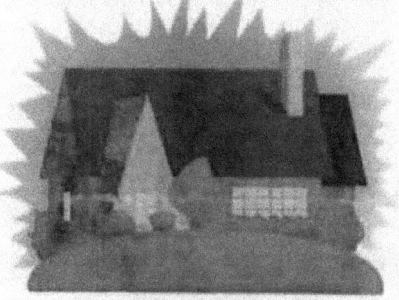

Residential
Commercial
Construction

For more information call Betty Scott

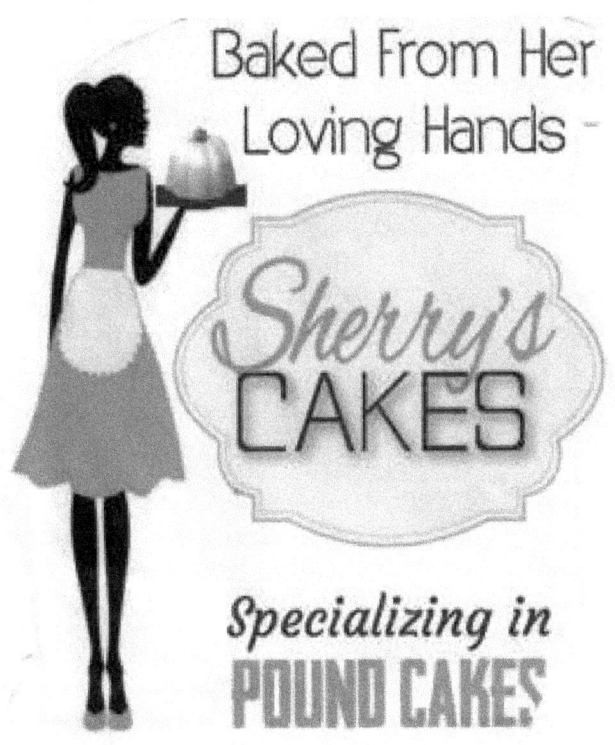

www.ingramcontent.com/pod-product-compliance
Lightning Source LLC
Chambersburg PA
CBHW070517090426
42735CB00012B/2822

Other Books and Series by Jeff Bowen

1901-1907 Native American Census Seneca, Eastern Shawnee, Miami, Modoc, Ottawa, Peoria, Quapaw, and Wyandotte Indians (Under Seneca School, Indian Territory)

1932 Census of The Standing Rock Sioux Reservation with Births And Deaths 1924-1932

Census of The Blackfeet, Montana, 1897- 1901 Expanded Edition

Eastern Cherokee by Blood, 1906-1910, Volumes I thru XIII

Choctaw of Mississippi Indian Census 1929-1932 with Births and Deaths 1924-1931   Volume I
Choctaw of Mississippi Indian Census 1933, 1934 & 1937, Supplemental Rolls to 1934 & 1935 with Births and Deaths 1932-1938, and Marriages 1936-1938 Volume II

Eastern Cherokee Census Cherokee, North Carolina 1930-1939 Census 1930-1931 with Births And Deaths 1924-1931 Taken By Agent L. W. Page Volume I
Eastern Cherokee Census Cherokee, North Carolina 1930-1939 Census 1932-1933 with Births And Deaths 1930-1932 Taken By Agent R. L. Spalsbury   Volume II
Eastern Cherokee Census Cherokee, North Carolina 1930-1939 Census 1934-1937 with Births and Deaths 1925-1938 and Marriages 1936 & 1938 Taken by Agents R. L. Spalsbury And Harold W. Foght Volume III

Seminole of Florida Indian Census, 1930-1940 with Birth and Death Records, 1930-1938

Texas Cherokees 1820-1839 A Document For Litigation 1921

Choctaw By Blood Enrollment Cards 1898-1914 Volumes I thru XVII

Starr Roll 1894 (Cherokee Payment Rolls) Districts: Canadian, Cooweescoowee, and Delaware Volume One
Starr Roll 1894 (Cherokee Payment Rolls) Districts: Flint, Going Snake, and Illinois   Volume Two
Starr Roll 1894 (Cherokee Payment Rolls) Districts: Saline, Sequoyah, and Tahlequah; Including Orphan Roll   Volume Three

Cherokee Intruder Cases Dockets of Hearings 1901-1909 Volumes I & II

Indian Wills, 1911-1921 Records of the Bureau of Indian Affairs Books One thru Seven;
Native American Wills & Probate Records 1911-1921

Other Books and Series by Jeff Bowen

Turtle Mountain Reservation Chippewa Indians 1932 Census with Births & Deaths, 1924-1932

Chickasaw By Blood Enrollment Cards 1898-1914 Volume I thru V

Cherokee Descendants East An Index to the Guion Miller Applications Volume I
Cherokee Descendants West An Index to the Guion Miller Applications Volume II (A-M)
Cherokee Descendants West An Index to the Guion Miller Applications Volume III (N-Z)

Applications for Enrollment of Seminole Newborn Freedmen, Act of 1905

Eastern Cherokee Census, Cherokee, North Carolina, 1915-1922, Taken by Agent James E. Henderson   *Volume I (1915-1916)*
                                    Volume II (1917-1918)
                                    Volume III (1919-1920)
                                    Volume IV (1921-1922)

Complete Delaware Roll of 1898

Eastern Cherokee Census, Cherokee, North Carolina, 1923-1929, Taken by Agent James E. Henderson   *Volume I (1923-1924)*
                                    Volume II (1925-1926)
                                    Volume III (1927-1929)

Applications for Enrollment of Seminole Newborn Act of 1905 Volumes I & II

North Carolina Eastern Cherokee Indian Census 1898-1899, 1904, 1906, 1909-1912, 1914 Revised and Expanded Edition

1932 Hopi and Navajo Native American Census with Birth & Death Rolls (1925-1931) Volume 1 - Hopi
1932 Hopi and Navajo Native American Census with Birth & Death Rolls (1930-1932) Volume 2 - Navajo

Western Navajo Reservation Navajo, Hopi and Paiute 1933 Census with Birth & Death Rolls 1925-1933

Cherokee Citizenship Commission Dockets 1880-1884 and 1887-1889 Volumes I thru V

Applications for Enrollment of Chickasaw Newborn Act of 1905 Volumes I & II

Visit our website at **www.nativestudy.com** to learn more about these and other books and series by Jeff Bowen